get your smile on:

Finally, Refreshing Answers
to Your Biggest Dental Questions!

Dr. Steve Thompson DDS, MAGD

Master of the Academy of General Dentistry

ISBN: 1453866507
ISBN-13: 9781453866504

Table of Contents

* Get your free bonus chapter by going online to
www.GetYourSmileOnBook.com/bonus-chapter

Introduction:

Get Your Smile On!

As a practicing master dentist with a busy office in Plano, Texas, I get asked a lot of questions:

- "Will this hurt?"
- "How badly will this hurt?"
- "What's that big shiny thing in your hand? And will it hurt me?"
- "How long will it hurt me?"

All kidding aside, I've always been concerned about those big issue questions patients *weren't* asking me about! You know the kind (you may even have some of your own)—those big ticket items that people dwell on, worry about, and mull over for years before perhaps summoning up the courage to come to me and ask.

For instance, there's a very poignant testimonial on my Web site from a great guy who waited years before approaching me about a certain dental issue. Well, here, I'll let him tell it:

"I finally got the nerve up to ask Dr. Thompson if he could straighten my teeth. He agreed...I was happy with what they looked like after the first four months. I'm glad that I found someone who is as precise and as encouraging as Dr. Thompson has been to me..." —C. B.

Unfortunately, guys like C.B. and plenty of my other patients wait way too long to approach me about these very serious issues. I know it's not their fault. Let's face it: people don't exactly jump for joy when it comes time to consider their teeth.

So I decided to take it upon myself and Google to find the most **popular, concerned with,** and **asked about** topics relating to dental health on the web. Here is what I found:

Checkups and Cleanings: Even if you take great care of your teeth, you still need regular checkups and cleanings. During this visit there are many critical items that must be accomplished that most people are not aware of and that many dentists overlook! For example, cavities and periodontal disease do not often exhibit symptoms until serious damage has been done, resulting in the need for expensive and often painful dental procedures. What's more, research has shown that gum disease (a symptom of irregular, infrequent, or skipped cleanings) can lead to a host of major health problems such as an increased risk for heart disease, heart attack, stroke, pancreatic cancer, Alzheimer's, low birth weight babies, etc. Don't know what you should be getting at your cleaning appointment? Never fear: I'll tell you what you should ask for!

Treating TMJ: People with age-worn smiles, bad bites, headaches, and TMJ pain (temporomandibular joint disorder) often suffer needlessly for years before seeking treatment. You don't have to suffer another minute after I explain all about TMJ therapy, which helps restore the natural health, bite, comfort, and beauty of your smile using nature as our treatment model. In a healthy and comfortable smile, the teeth, jaw joints, and muscles are functioning together in harmony.

Sedation Dentistry: "I want to have healthy teeth but I am afraid and embarrassed by my fear. Is there a way that you can help me?" It's a question I hear quite often and one that, finally, there *is* an answer for. Did you know that the biggest reason why most people fear, put off, or completely avoid getting various dental procedures done is because they have a great deal of anxiety over the kind of pain they may experience while in a dental chair? Sedation dentistry is the perfect solution for most patients who suffer from dental anxiety. Sedation dentistry can make your next dental visit more relaxing, more comfortable, and anxiety free. It can literally change your life!

Cosmetic Dentistry: Patients often come to me after suffering for years from pain, insecurity, or lack of confidence over their facial features. Cosmetic dentistry, Botox, and Juvederm are about more than making you beautiful; they're about making you feel beautiful—inside and out.

Dental Implants: Dental implants are modern science's way of replacing weakened teeth or missing teeth with long-lasting solutions. The implant is used as a support, or base, into which new teeth, multiple new teeth, or dentures are attached. Imagine being able to rely on strong, fixed, and permanent teeth again for chewing or talking with pride. For those patients who are insecure about missing or rotting teeth, implants can improve not only your appearance but your confidence as well, as old insecurities become a thing of the past. Everything you ever wanted to know about dental implants but were afraid to ask will be answered in *Get Your Smile On!*

All About Invisalign: These days, there are a variety of ways to improve the appearance of your teeth without braces. One such method is Invisalign®, designed to straighten your teeth. Removable, clear Invisalign provides patients with a revolutionary way to straighten teeth without the limitations of traditional braces. Now, you can choose to improve the look and function of your teeth with flexible, removable Invisalign aligners.

Botox and Dermal Fillers: The safe and noninvasive way to have fuller lips and a younger face and smile in a matter of minutes. Go online to www.GetYourSmileOnBook.com/bonus-chapter to receive your bonus chapter, "Are Dermal Fillers and Botox Right for You?"

Now that I know what my patients are most interested in, I wanted to write it all down so *all* dental patients—everywhere—

could have something to smile about. So if you're ready to *Get Your Smile On*, the answers to these burning dental questions await.

Chapter 1:

Checkups and Cleanings

Once upon a time, you went to the dentist twice a year, got your teeth cleaned, a free toothbrush sample with the doctor's name on it, and that was that. (Maybe, if you were lucky, some free toothpaste thrown in as well!) But that was then and this is now. New research indicates that regular dental cleanings, periodic checkups, and all-around careful dental care doesn't just affect the way you smile—it could just save your life.

Now more than ever, people are at risk for letting their mouths go by the wayside. When times are tight, as they have been for most of us recently, dental cleanings and regular checkups are one of the first things to be let go from the family budget.

What's more, over-the-counter cleaning systems and pricey toothpastes promise whiter and stronger teeth, cleaner gums, less oral bacteria, and fresher breath, so people feel as if they can skip the dentist altogether as long as their teeth aren't hurting, turning yellow, and people don't cringe whenever they speak. But there is more to oral health care than clean teeth and fresh breath.

Even if you take great care of your teeth, you still need regular checkups and cleanings. During this visit there are many critical items that must be accomplished that most people are not aware of—and that many dentists overlook!

What Happens During a Routine Cleaning and Checkup?

A Imagecare Dental we practice what we call, "Patient Centered Dentistry" where the focus is on the patients I think it's important for patients to know not just what we're doing during a "routine" checkup and cleaning but *why* we're doing it as well.

For instance, we are doing more than merely polishing their teeth. In fact, we are performing the following four critical steps:

Step 1—Routine Dental Checkup: Anything But Routine!

Believe it or not, there is actually nothing routine about your dental checkup/exam. While most patients assume that they are there to simply get their teeth cleaned, much more happens during this visit.

In fact, if no other dentist has told you already, let me be the first to say that a trip to the dentist's chair is no different from a trip to the doctor's office for your yearly physical. In fact, let me be the first to go so far as to call this a routine physical—for your mouth.

That's actually what it is. Research has discovered that a host of ills—including diabetes, heart disease, cancer, and even Alzheimer's—can be linked back to poor dental care or oral bacteria, and so what I'm actually doing is giving your mouth a routine physical. Here's what I'm checking for when I ask you to "open wide":

Soft Tissue Exam: I do a careful analysis of the various "soft tissues" present within the mouth, checking for the following:
- Growths, masses, oral cancer, disease, or blocked salivary glands, swollen lymph nodes, and swollen tonsils
- Saliva consistency and salivary flow

Periodontal Exam: Periodontal is another word for "gum," and that is the region I am specifically examining during this part of the checkup. We perform a full periodontal probing each visit and compare to previous visits. Here, in particular, is what I'm looking for:
- Periodontal disease
- Gingivitis
- Plaque and calculus levels
- Inflammation and ulcerative conditions

Bite Exam: Your "bite" is determined by how your teeth come together, or align. It can be affected by the wear upon your teeth from chewing, grinding, and possible misalignment, which can lead to headaches or even chronic TMJ pain. Here is what I'm looking for in this exam:

- Tooth alignment
- Tooth wear
- TMJ pain, popping, or clicking
- Jaw muscle pain
- Soft tissue evidence of clenching or grinding, such as scalloping of the tongue, sloughing tissue on the sides of your cheek, or gum recession
- Common or recurring headaches (which can mean jaw misalignment or even chronic TMJ pain)

Tooth-by-tooth Exam: In this critical exam I literally go tooth-by-tooth and evaluate the following:

- Tooth disease or infection
- Integrity of existing restorations
- Cavities, abscesses, and fractures in teeth

Esthetic Exam: What do your teeth look like? This is the type of thing I look for in the Esthetic Exam. Other items I look for include:

- Esthetics of teeth and gums
- Tooth color
- Rotated and chipped teeth

Clearly, a checkup is more than just a cleaning and a cleaning is more than just a checkup. Again, if you begin to think of a trip to your dentist's office in the same way you do a trip to any other doctor's office, you'll not only take these visits more seriously but follow recommendations more closely.

Step 2—Ultra Sonic: Bring Your Towel!

Plaque is a buildup of bacteria, food debris, and bacteria byproducts that results over time. Even the best toothbrushes and most expensive toothpastes, water picks, and electric brushes can't remove all the plaque that resides on your teeth.

Why? Because not all of your tooth is visible or able to be reached by over-the-counter methods. Unremoved plaque will begin to calcify or harden and become what's known as "calculus" or tartar. The buildup of plaque and calculus on teeth is home to millions of bacteria and if left for too long can migrate down in between the tooth and gums causing gingivitis (inflammation of the gums), which can progress to periodontal disease.

Removal of the plaque and calculus is a critical phase of your routine cleaning. Remember those sharp but precise, long, metal instruments and the ultrasonic scaler that shoots water everywhere? (That's what you need the towel for!) They are used to scale away the plaque and calculus from your teeth.

For most people, six months is the appropriate interval between cleaning and checkups, but for some a more frequent visit is necessary due to higher levels of accumulation, gingivitis, gum disease or a past history of gum disease, tooth crowding, lack of flossing, or during pregnancy.

Step 3—Polishing: The Flavored Grit!

Polishing the patient's teeth is more than just a cosmetic part of the routine; here is an additional opportunity to clean away any remaining plaque buildup leftover from the scaling portion of the cleaning. This gives you the nice, smooth, clean feeling.

Plus you get to choose your flavor. Fun!

Step 4—Fluoride Treatments: Dentistry's Magic "Silver Bullet"

What if there was a magical, natural "silver bullet" that could prevent tooth decay, strengthen teeth, and help you avoid cavities and painful and expensive dental procedures all in one?

There is: it's called fluoride. Most dentists and researchers agree: if it weren't for fluoride, dentists would be working overtime all across the country just to keep up with America's fillings!

Once upon a time, we were taught that only children needed fluoride treatments beyond the water they drank and the toothpaste they used; now we know better. In fact, Surgeon General Richard H. Carmona insists that "Fluoridation is the single most effective public health measure to prevent tooth decay and improve oral health over a lifetime, for both children *and adults*."

And, according to WebMD.com, "New research indicates that topical fluoride—from toothpastes, mouth rinses, and **fluoride treatments**—are as important in fighting tooth decay as in strengthening developing teeth."

Why is fluoride so important? The answer lies in cavities, but it's much more serious than you think. Once a cavity gets too big or extends to the root of the tooth, it's like the "beginning of the end" of that tooth. How do we prevent this from happening? Unfortunately, once you have a root cavity, there is usually no predictable cure; we drill it and fill it to the best of our ability and hope for the best. No, the only way to "cure" a root cavity is to avoid it in the first place. And how do we do that? That's right, with fluoride.

The good news is that most dentists include some type of fluoride treatment as an integral part of their routine cleaning and maintenance. Now, if you're an adult who remembers the old school fluoride treatments, which were bitter and acidic, you're probably greeting this newsflash with a frown. But here's the good news: not only do our modern fluoride treatments come in great-tasting new flavors like mint and bubble gum, but they last just about sixty seconds—or less!

So if your dentist doesn't make a fluoride treatment part of your regular exam, insist on it—or go elsewhere. Your teeth are too important to leave to chance; and remember, once you get a cavity, it's too late!

Step 5—Assessment and Recommendations

Finally, the fifth component of a routine checkup and cleaning procedure is to make a valid assessment of what I've just seen and recommendations for further treatment.

For instance, if I've noticed excessively red and recessed gums from aggressive brushing, I may suggest using a soft toothbrush or a Sonicare toothbrush. If I've spotted a potential cavity or looming periodontal disease, I may recommend a filling or periodontal therapy for gum infection.

Recommendations can be as simple as "brush once more a day with a soft brush" to a more complex prescription for dental implants or a bridge. Regardless of what we find during a routine checkup and cleaning, our goal for you is simple: to correct any present problems we may have uncovered during the exam, prevent future problems, and provide you with an accurate prioritized roadmap back to ideal health.

It is very important that your dentist be up front and honest about your needs. Overlooking or delaying problems in your mouth can often lead to more problems, distrust in your dentist, and a feeling like you're needing more work every time you come into the office (a "nickel and dimed to death" mentality that often discourages patients from coming back).

Remember, your dentist is not the enemy; he or she is there to see to all of your oral needs—past, present, and future. Finding the right dentist is often the first step in taking better care of your teeth and gums.

If Your Tooth Already Hurts, It's Too Late for a "Routine" Dental Visit

You know how they say if you're thirsty, your body is already dehydrated? Well, if your tooth already hurts, you've already gone beyond a "routine" dental visit. The fact of the matter is that dental pain is a sign of more than just too much candy or not enough fluoride.

Here is a list of common dental complaints and what they might mean:

- **Sore, bleeding or enflamed gums:** Any of these indicators—sore, bleeding or inflamed gums—could be signs of gingivitis or gum disease.
- **Receding gums:** Gums that have receded—i.e. pulled away from the teeth—could indicate advanced gum disease, bone loss, and bite problems.
- **Tooth sensitivity:** Sensitive teeth can mean that the enamel on your teeth has been worn down, typically due to an acidic diet and/or lack of proper dental care. A tooth that hurts when eating or one that is sensitive to hot and cold temperatures could mean you have a cracked tooth, a cavity or need a root canal.
- **Halitosis (bad breath):** Sometimes we get bad breath from what we eat, while other times bad breath can be a sign of more serious dental issues like a cavity or even gingivitis—or gum disease. But in other cases halitosis—or bad breath—which persists can be indicative of more serious health issues like a sinus infection, a yeast infection, gastric reflux, or even diabetes.

Clean Now, Not Later

Of course, every dentist makes it a point to make sure you come for a checkup twice a year, but have you ever stopped to wonder why? It's because we know that it's not what you can see on your teeth or even feel in your mouth or smell on your breath that counts, but what that seeing, feeling, and smelling mean.

For example, cavities and periodontal disease do not often exhibit symptoms until serious damage has been done, resulting in the need for expensive and often painful dental procedures.

It's just like taking care of your vehicle. If you never change your oil, how can you expect your car to last more than one hundred thousand miles? And if you never get the factory recommended maintenance, how can you get mad at the car mechanic for telling you the transmission needs to be replaced—for $2,500?

Every day I have to tell smart, capable, intelligent, organized people that they have a cavity, that they might need a root canal, that one or more teeth are going to come out, and that it was all *preventable.*

There is nothing more frustrating to the modern dentist than having to fill or extract teeth because of simple neglect. And that's what it is: neglect. A good toothbrush costs a buck or two; ditto for dental floss. Even a really, really good toothpaste only costs three or four bucks.

And while dental visits are slightly more expensive, major dental issues can cost five and even ten times as much as a cleaning and checkup if you let things go for too long. But it's not just dollars and cents at risk here. As you're about to see, what happens in and around the mouth often leads to—or can at least indicate—the overall health of the rest of your body.

A Question of Cavities

Some of the most common questions I get are about cavities. And of all the cavity questions I get, this one is the *most* common: "Doctor, why didn't you find that cavity during my last visit six months ago?" Another version of the question from our new patients is "Why didn't my *last* dentist find these cavities?"

First of all, let me say that this is an excellent question and one that any good dentist will be able to answer for you. Did you know that cavities form from bacterial byproducts (i.e., acid) dissolving the tooth structure? In fact, this is why most cavities occur in areas that are neglected or hard to reach.

Bacteria-laden plaque fueled by carbohydrates (i.e. sugars) drive this process. Cavities start out microscopic in nature and progressively grow over time until they are detectable. By the time they are visible on the X-ray or by the dental explorer, you can know that the cavity has been there for quite some time; it was merely undetectable until now.

Eventually, the cavity gets to the point that it is detectable by your dentist. Of course, the smart aleck side of me wants to say in response to this question, "Well, if I had detected the cavity six months ago at your last visit, you would have asked me the same question, then likewise six months prior to that and on and on. Cavities have to become detectable at some point!"

So to avoid being a smart aleck, I will instead share with you that one of the best ways I have found to answer this question is by using a timeline followed by an explanation of cavities by comparing them to a disease that most people are more familiar with: cancer.

First up, the timeline:

Cavity Timeline

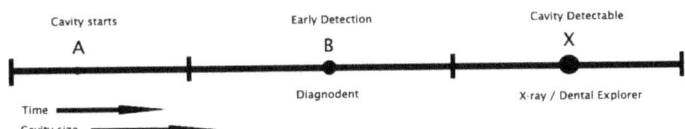

On our timeline above, a cavity starts at point A and grows. Its rate of growth varies. This growth rate is affected by many factors, such as your diet, saliva pH, and oral hygiene habits! So as time goes by, this microscopic cavity grows larger and larger until we reach point X on the timeline. At last, *this* is the point at which the cavity is detectible by the dental explorer or X-rays.

Voila, now you have a detectable cavity! So, the answer to the question is simple: **The cavity was not detectable at your last visit**. Regardless if your last visit was one year ago, six months ago, or six weeks ago, the answer is the same: it wasn't detectable! So, your next question is probably something like this: "You mean to tell me that a cavity that was previously undetectable six months ago is now detectable?" That's exactly what I mean! At some point on the timeline most cavities become detectable.

Now, let's move on to my cancer analogy. First of all, let me say that tooth decay is *not* cancer and you will likely *not* die from tooth decay—but the two *do* behave similarly. Just like point A on our cavity timeline, where decay starts, cancer starts.

It may be months or years before you have any symptoms, and even then, sometimes symptoms may precede your diagnosis because the cancer is not yet detectable. Thankfully, modern medicine has advanced to where we can diagnose cancer much earlier than ever before. Years ago, all we had to rely on were symptoms, X-rays, and exploratory surgery; but now with MRIs, CT scans, and ultrasound, we can catch cancer much sooner.

Now, let me jump back to our cavity timeline for just a minute. You may have noticed point B on the timeline. Not only do we have and routinely use a CT scanner in our office, now many dental offices that stay up with technology are equipped with a laser cavity detector called a Diagnodent.

This advanced device allows us to detect decay much earlier than ever before, and with a greater degree of accuracy than any method used in the past. It represents a quantum leap forward in our diagnostic capabilities. Everybody knows how important it is to treat cancer early, especially before it metastasizes to other parts of the body. Likewise, it is important to treat cavities as early as possible before they destroy healthy tissues, spread to other locations in the mouth, or even cause death to the tooth.

Just like early detection is the key to surviving cancer, early cavity detection is critical to saving your tooth. Bear with me as I stretch this cancer analogy a little further to make one last point.

Let's suppose you went in for an age-recommend colonoscopy (whoopee!) and your doctor found a cancerous polyp. Now, prior to this diagnosis you had no symptoms, no pain, and were otherwise healthy. Would you say to your doctor, "Hey, Doc, this thing doesn't hurt, it's not bothering me, so I don't want to have it treated"? No, you wouldn't say that at all. Instead, you would say, "Hey, get that cancerous polyp out of there as soon as you can before spreads!"

Again, cavities are usually not life threatening, but you should have the same mentality toward a cavity as you do toward cancer! Take care of it early, take care of it now, so no more damage occurs and your tooth stays alive, strong, and healthy.

Your Mouth—A Gateway to Health (Or Ills)

Research has shown that gum disease (cause by improper home care or irregular, infrequent, or skipped cleanings) can lead to a host of major health problems such as an increased risk for heart disease, heart attack, stroke, pancreatic cancer, Alzheimer's, low birth weight babies, etc.

According to the American Academy of Periodontology, "Research has shown, and experts agree, that there is an association between periodontal diseases and other chronic inflammatory conditions, such as diabetes, cardiovascular disease, and Alzheimer's disease. Therefore, treating inflammation may not only help manage periodontal diseases but may also help with the management of other chronic inflammatory conditions."

Sheila Wolf, RDH, author of *Pregnancy and Oral Health*, agrees. "Gum disease, a chronic bacterial infection, affects nearly 75 percent of the general population at one time or another. These chronic infections have been linked to increased risk of heart attack, stroke, ulcers, diabetes, respiratory diseases, and pregnancy complications."

Clearly, your mouth is linked to your overall health. This means bad breath can be a sign of mere halitosis, or something inside your body crying to be found out. It also means inflamed gums can be signs of a greater infection somewhere else in the body.

No longer is a checkup merely a checkup! Instead, it is a routine physical—of your mouth!

Five Things You Should Ask Your Dentist During a Cleaning or Checkup

Don't know what you should be getting at your cleaning appointment? Never fear: I'll tell you what you should ask for! First and foremost, make sure you understand everything that is being said. If you ask a question and get "doctor speak" in reply, ask again; ask until you get an answer that makes sense to you.

Next, make sure you know what's going to be happening to you—and why. I've explained the five segments of our patient centered routine with every patient, but maybe your dentist is different. If so, ask why.

More specifically, here are the five things you (and every patient) should ask at the dentist during a cleaning or checkup:

1.) What, exactly, are you going to be doing today?
2.) Is there anything I need to understand better about the treatment you recommended?
3.) Doc, please show me the X-rays and intraoral camera pictures so I can be involved in my own treatment plan.
4.) What could I have done from a preventative standpoint on my own to keep my mouth healthier?
5.) Is there anything I need to do in advance for my next visit?

Parting Words about Checkups and Cleanings

By now you probably know more than you ever did—or even wanted to know—about your routine checkups and cleanings. Great! That's why I'm here. The fact is that unless you read medical journals or go to dental school, you might not know that periodontal disease is related to heart disease or that serious problems can develop without feeling pain. Routine preventative dental care could save your life.

We need to stop thinking of dentistry as a "when" scenario. In other words, when you have the money, when you have the time, or worst of all, when you have a toothache!

Regular cleanings, home health care, and a general attitude of oral health need to go hand-in-hand to create not just happier and healthier patients but happier and healthier mouths as well.

Chapter 2:

Treating TMJ

Have you had headaches or jaw pain for the past few weeks?
The past few months?
Even the past few years?
Advil may help a little, but it's merely a bandage, not a cure.

You may have even tried more traditional methods like visiting your doctor or a chiropractor, or maybe you've even tried acupuncture, herbalists, or other less traditional means—yet nothing helps.

The fact of the matter is that headaches and jaw pain are just one of the many symptoms of something known as TMJ, or temporomandibular joint disorder, and if this is the case going to regular doctor, a chiropractor, or even an acupuncturist likely won't be a long-term solution. But going to your dentist will.

What Is a Temporomandibular Joint?

In the human body, joints are known as the intersection between crucial muscles, bones, or tendons. Your jaw is no different. Cushioned by a disc, the temporomandibular joint (TMJ) helps keep the lower jaw connected to the skull.

The TMJ joint is actually one of the most complex joints in the body due to its wide range of movements and the fact that it has to work in harmony with another set of structures, the teeth.

The symptoms of TMJ disorder are not limited to only jaw pain; there are a number of other symptoms, which can include:

- Tinnitus (ringing in the ears)
- Loose teeth
- Facial pain

- Clicking/popping of the jaw
- Limited jaw movement/locking jaw
- Worn/cracked teeth
- Not being unable to open the mouth comfortably
- Headaches
- A bite that feels uncomfortable or "off"
- Neck, shoulder, and back pain
- Swelling on the side of the face
- Fullness or a sense of pressure in your ear

Are you experiencing any of these additional symptoms? If so, you may have TMJ. The good news is twofold: first, you're not alone and second—there *is* help for you.

You Are Not Alone: *Treatment for TMJ*

According to Dentistry.com, "An estimated ten million Americans suffer from TMJ disorders."

Jaw pain can be one the most uncomfortable feelings in the world. Not only is it painful, but it also limits so many enjoyable things in life: eating, socializing, sleeping, and many others. Many people simply ignore jaw pain. Some deal with the pain with pain-killers. Others wait for it to go away.

If you have been experiencing jaw pain, there is help for you. Before I explain more, let me ask you a few questions. **In addition to jaw pain, do you suffer from one or any of these symptoms?**

- Headaches and migraines?
- Neck and shoulder pain?
- Bad bite?
- Sensitive or sore teeth?
- Teeth and dental restorations that are worn flat or cracking?

If you answered yes, we may have already identified your problem. You may have something called TMJ.

TMJ, the short-form of temporomandibular joint syndrome, also known as temporomandibular joint disorder (TMD) is easily one of the least understood and most under-diagnosed oral conditions. This is quite a surprising fact considering that there are well over ten million TMJ sufferers in the United States alone!

What Causes TMJ?

The primary cause of TMJ is disharmony between the jaw (TMJ) and the position of the teeth. As a result many people tend to grind their teeth, which is the brain's attempt to achieve harmony.

There are a variety of other causes, some physical, some emotional. For instance, stressful behavior and emotional times in our lives can lead to a conscious and later unconscious grinding of our teeth (known as "bruxism").

This teeth grinding can occur during the day when we're not fully conscious of it (it's easier to spot this behavior in others than it is in ourselves) and then continue on at night while we sleep.

An injury to the face, neck, or head—or even to the temporomandibular joint itself—can obviously affect how this sensitive joint operates and create pain, frustration, and a feeling of helplessness in the sufferer. If teeth are missing or poorly aligned, this can cause an improper bite that over time can weaken, damage, or otherwise affect the temporomandibular joint and cause pain and suffering as well.

Unfortunately, many people with age-worn smiles, bad bites, headaches, and TMJ pain often suffer needlessly for years before seeking treatment.

You don't have to suffer another minute! Imagecare TMJ therapy helps restore the natural health, bite, comfort, and beauty of your smile using nature as our treatment model. In a healthy and comfortable smile, the teeth, jaw joints, and muscles are functioning together in harmony.

Unfortunately, TMJ Doesn't Just "Go Away"

It is vital to know that your TMJ symptoms won't simply remain as they are. Although TMJ symptoms ebb and flow, they are typically progressive, and that means they will get worse over time. Furthermore, as time goes by, you may suffer from an increasing number of symptoms, and as the symptoms worsen, they can actually cause real damage to your TMJ joint such as displacement of the joint disc or tear in the disc.

Left untreated, you may suffer from significant pain in the head, neck, and shoulder region, not just in your facial area. Many times, people suffering from these pains don't have any idea that the cause is in their jaw. They may have seen many doctors, from ENTs to neurologists, with no results that can lead to proper treatment.

By being checked by a dentist that specializes in TMJ, you may discover that the issue was in your jaw all along, and that treatment can begin right away. Until you receive your treatment, it is recommended that you take the following steps to assist in managing your symptoms and reducing any pain:

- Take a non-aspirin pain reliever or a muscle relaxant, anti-inflammatory drug, or analgesic.
- Use Imagecare TMJ Physical therapy guide.
- Avoid chewing gum.
- Eat soft foods.
- Apply ice or moist heat.
- Practice relaxation techniques that minimize muscle tension.
- Practice good stress management techniques.
- Keep good posture.
- Relax and keep teeth apart.

How Can I Just Get Rid of the Pain?

First, you need a proper diagnosis before you begin treatment. This means going to a dentist that deals with TMJ issues on a regular basis. The sooner you receive a proper diagnosis, the sooner you can begin to relieve all of the symptoms that you're feeling, and make sure that the symptoms do not progress into more serious problems.

This will likely involve a multifaceted treatment plan.

I find people who have healthy, stable joints; proper tooth guidance; and proper tooth form to be more attractive and youthful and have less orthodontic relapse, joint problems, periodontal (gum) problems, TMJ pain or TMJ dysfunction (TMD), pain, and/ or tooth wear. People in general are becoming more aware of problems like these and are seeking solutions. Imagecare TMJ Therapy can help solve these problems.

When we feel pain in our teeth, our gums, or even our jaws, the obvious first choice is to visit a dentist. Unfortunately, not all dentists are created equal. Some just handle basic problems, while others actually do handle TMJ cases and are quite good at it.

The problem is that few dentists will turn away a TMJ patient, whether they know how to treat it effectively or not. Most, in fact, have good intentions; they assume that there must be some kind of pressure or misalignment causing the pain and that by simply relieving the pressure or forcing realignment, the pain will go away.

Unfortunately, this is not always the case. Making lasting, permanent, and often significant changes to the alignment of the teeth and, in essence, the very shape of the mouth can do more harm than good if not performed by a highly trained dentist.

Imagecare TMJ Therapy answers this call by using nature and science to our best advantage. Our TMJ therapy is based on principles taught by the OBI Foundation for Bioesthetic Dentistry founded by Dr Bob Lee.

The Imagecare Smile

An Imagecare Smile is a naturally beautiful smile that appears youthful, has normal biologic form free from wear, has normal function, and is comfortable.

When you look closely at an Imagecare Smile, you see a smile that is attractive. You see how teeth overlap and fit together. You will also see each front tooth is of an appropriate length and the back teeth have well-defined anatomy, especially the cuspids (canines). What you don't see is poorly aligned teeth, worn or missing teeth, and tense facial muscles. This natural biologic tooth form is found in the absence of dental malocclusion and bite dysfunction.

The significance of an Imagecare Smile is not only how it appears but also, and more importantly, **how it functions**. Each tooth has a genetic biologic form that determines its function in helping your teeth and jaws to chew correctly. Smiles that have worn or misaligned teeth cannot function properly, and when not functioning properly can lead to disharmony between TMJ and teeth, leading to TMJ dysfunction.

Many people are unaware that they may have a bite disharmony or dysfunction, but exhibit some of the signs and symptoms anyway. Like heart disease or diabetes, many of the early signs and symptom of bite dysfunction go undetected for many years while damage is occurring because the symptoms seem unrelated to a bite problem. For a very good video demonstration of what TMJ function might look like, go to www.imagecaredentalgroup.com/plano-tmj-dentist.html.

Do I Have Bite Dysfunction?

If you have an attractive smile, unworn teeth, and are pain free, you most likely have a healthy smile. If you have any of the following signs pictured in the figure below, chances are you may have a bite dysfunction and the health of your mouth, teeth. and jaws are at risk.

Bite Dysfunction Self-test

If you are experiencing one or more of these signs and symptoms, chances are that a problem is present. Ignoring these problems can lead to irreversible damage of your teeth, gums and jaw joints.

- Worn teeth
- Cracked or broken teeth
- Sore of stiff jaw muscles
- Facial pain
- Pain with chewing
- Loose teeth
- Clenching or grinding of teeth
- Receding gums

- Abfractions (notching of the teeth at gum line)
- Uncomfortable bite
- Shifting teeth or bite
- Jaw clicking or popping
- TMJ pain/TMD (temporomandibular dysfunction)

If I Have Bite Dysfunction, What Should I Do?

If you are experiencing any of the signs or symptoms presented in this chapter, a comprehensive bite analysis is needed to evaluate your chewing system. To accurately diagnose a bite dysfunction or TMJ problems, mounted study models of your teeth are essential along with a dental examination, periodontal examination, jaw joint evaluation, and muscle examination.

The models of your teeth are then mounted on an instrument (articulator) that simulates your lower jaw movements allowing the dentist to evaluate the mechanics of your bite in relation to your jaw joints. Once the problem is identified, a solution to restore harmony to your chewing system can be discussed.

How Is Bite Dysfunction Corrected?

After a comprehensive diagnosis is completed, restoring harmony to your chewing system to correct the bite dysfunction is unique to your specific problem. There are three treatment goals to correct bite dysfunction and restore your smile:

1. **Stable jaw joints (TMJs):** The jaw joints are properly positioned.

2. **Proper tooth form:** All teeth exhibit proper unworn anatomy and touch simultaneously when jaw joints are properly rotated to a closed mouth position.

3. **Anterior guidance:** The front teeth guide the lower jaw movements, protecting the back teeth from colliding abnormally during normal chewing motions.

In most cases, a specialized appliance called a Maxillary Anterior Guided Orthosis (MAGO) is used to locate a stable position for your jaw joints, satisfying the first treatment goal. Meeting the second and third goals requires definitive solutions that may include bite adjustments, bonding, braces, crowns, and in some worst-case scenarios, jaw surgery.

In some cases, a combination of treatment is required to correct the imbalance in the chewing system so the teeth, bones, muscles, and joints can work properly together. The result is a long-lasting, comfortable, naturally attractive Imagecare Smile of your own. If you are suffering from any of the effects of bite dysfunction listed above, including TMJ pain, you need a TMJ dentist who can help you!

Chapter 3:

Sedation Dentistry

Making regular visits to your dentist is one of the best ways to preserve the health of your teeth and to prevent future, more extensive dental procedures. For many people, it's simple to schedule their twice-yearly dental visits and make the best of them. Like routine auto maintenance, it's a fact of life and they go whether they're looking forward to it or not.

For some patients, however, the thought of going to the dentist creates a great deal of anxiety; in fact, some people are so fearful of going to a dentist that they simply never go, which only causes their dental problems to worsen.

Imagine simply *not* going to the dentist. Not because you can't afford it, not because your teeth don't hurt, not because you don't know that you need to, but because you're simply too afraid to pick up the phone and make that appointment.

Now there is a new form of dentistry that has made going to the dentist a bearable, if not pleasant experience, for the millions of people who have avoided the dentist for years and years. No longer do people need to be afraid of going to the dentist.

Sedation dentistry (sometimes referred to as sleep dentistry) just may be the answer you've been looking for to alleviate the fear and anxiety you experience just thinking about sitting in your dentist's chair.

Sedation dentistry is the perfect solution for most patients who suffer from dental anxiety. Imagine eliminating the fear from dentistry and making a trip to the dentist that is no more anxiety inducing than a trip to the movies or a ball game. Sedation dentistry options can make your next dental visit more relaxing, more comfortable, and anxiety free.

If You're Afraid of Going to the Dentist, Take Heart: *You Are Not Alone*

Believe it or not, millions of Americans have some form anxiety concerning dental treatment. This anxiety may range from very mild to severe. Some anxiety is so significant that it prevents necessary trips to the dental office.

This anxiety or fear coupled with embarrassment from years of neglect has kept almost half of the American population from seeking much needed dental treatment. The great news is that "dental phobia" is a thing of the past for many of these patients, who have discovered the secret to healthy teeth and a vibrant smile.

You may have noticed that modern dentists' offices have already responded to their patients' anxieties with spa-like amenities such as back massagers, laughing gas, warm towels/blankets, and soothing music. While these extra touches can certainly help take the edge off, to the extremely fearful patient these amenities are simply not enough.

For many patients, sedation dentistry has been an answer to their prayers! With conscious sedation, patients take two very safe, small pills about an hour before their appointment. These pills help patients feel extremely relaxed and help eliminate dental fear!

In fact, most patients feel so relaxed that they just snooze right through their appointment, pain-free, usually with no memory of the procedure. Often years of neglect are corrected in a single appointment without the need for IV sedation or general anesthesia. To many of these patients, this process is life changing.

Often these patients feel so relieved, it's almost like a burden or large obstacle was removed from their life. They get a new lease on life because this huge problem they've been facing is suddenly solved with two little pills.

Life is often busy and stressful and sedation dentistry can help you solve your dental problems so you can focus on changing the world (or, at the very least, your world). Sedation dentistry isn't for fearful patients only; it's also extremely helpful for patients requiring longer appointments just to make them more comfortable and relaxed.

What Is Sedation Dentistry?

According to Joseph De Avila writing on behalf of the *Wall Street Journal*:

> The [sedation dentistry] approach uses a variety of medications to bring about a state of conscious sedation, in which a patient isn't fully unconscious, but remains drowsy and only semi-aware during procedures.
>
> Dentists trained in the practice say the fastest-growing method involves oral sedatives such as Halcion, which they say offer more anxiety relief than nitrous oxide (aka laughing gas). And because temporary, short-term memory loss is a common side effect of these drugs, patients typically don't remember the experience.

Sedation dentistry isn't for everybody, but for the following types of patients it could just be the answer to their prayers:

- Patients who fear needles
- Patients who have difficulty becoming numb after local anesthetic
- Patients requiring multiple dental procedures
- Patients who have had bad past experiences at the dentist
- Patients who have a strong gag reflex
- Patients suffering from other physical disabilities
- Patients suffering from dental fear, anxiety, and embarrassment

Methods of Sedation

Dentists can use a number of medications to sedate their patients, and many patients assume sedation dentistry means they will absolutely be "asleep" during the procedure. However, that may not be the case. Some the most commonly used drugs to sedate dental patients are triazolam (Halcion), diazepam (Valium), lorazepam (Ativan) zaleoplon (Sonata), and hydroxyzine (Vistaril).

All of these medications have been proven to be safe and effective. Since all of these drugs work in different ways and last for different amounts of time, your certified sedation dentist will discuss the differences with you and decide which drug is most appropriate for the dental work you are having done that day.

Triazolam is the most popular choice because it actually has an amnesiac effect, and patients rarely remember what even happened at their appointment. This drug is especially effective for patients who are afraid of the dentist.

Some of these medications make patients drowsy enough that they will sleep through the procedure. For obvious reasons, being sedated before your dental procedures requires someone to drive you to and from the dentist's office.

How Does Sedation Dentistry Work?

Don't let the official name scare you off from going to the dentist anymore than you already have been. Sedation dentistry follows six simple steps to put your mind, and your body, at ease so that you can not only face going to the dentist without fear but hardly remember it after it's over:

- **Step 1**—*Making your first appointment*: This is difficult for many anxious people, so your dentist will naturally try to make this as easy as possible.
- **Step 2**—*Welcoming visit*: Next, your dentist will gather information regarding your health and discuss with you your wants and desires. If you're comfortable, your dentist will take X-rays and look in your mouth. But you will never be judged or embarrassed.
- **Step 3**—*Preparing for your sedation visit*: In Step 3, your dentist will give you a prescription for a sedative to take the night before your first appointment to guarantee a good night's sleep and to make sure you wake up relaxed.
- **Step 4**—*Arriving for treatment*: Your companion will bring you to the office. Additional medications will be provided to create the ultimate in relaxation. Your experienced sedation team will monitor you throughout your entire visit.

- **Step 5**—*Going home with your new smile*: Your companion will take you home and stay with you until you're completely recovered from your sedation medication.
- **Step 6**—*The next day*: Most patients feel no discomfort or residual effects, as by now the effects of sedation medications will have worn off. Instead, you will have a great feeling of accomplishment like a weight has been lifted, and you will be thrilled.

Seven Signs that Sedation Dentistry Might Be Right for You

Could sedation dentistry be the solution you've been looking for? Here are seven signs that sedation dentistry might be right for you:

1. **Delaying treatment you need and want?** As we have seen throughout this book, dental care is vital to your overall health. Don't think that brushing and flossing and whitening your teeth can replace your annual dental visits; they can't. Get treatment now, before it's too late.

2. **Scared, even terrified, to pick up the phone to schedule?** Some people have a genuine sense of anxiety when it comes to going to the dentist; others are literally terrified to go. What do these people do when they have a sore tooth, a cavity, or gingivitis? Sedation dentistry offers a viable alternative for those patients for whom anxiety is just the beginning of their feelings for going to the dentist.

3. **In pain, especially when you eat?** If your teeth are in pain, particularly when you're eating, it's a giant red flag that you need dental treatment. See what sedation dentistry can do for you.

4. **Someone who has trouble with gagging or getting numb?** Some of us have stronger gag reflexes than others, making a trip to the dentist excruciating torture when

asked *not* to gag. And if you're resistant to getting numb, dental procedures can take twice as long—and hurt twice as much. Sedation dentistry is a healthy, viable alternative for both types of patients.

5. **Having trouble finding someone you can trust?** The anxious or fearful dental patient often has a trouble in the cookie-cutter world of modern dentistry. Dentists like myself who specialize in sedation dentistry not only recognize this fear and anxiety but also know how to treat it—safely, patiently, and effectively.

6. **Looking to smile again with confidence?** If it's been awhile since you could smile with confidence, think of what sedation dentistry can do for you. Eliminating the fear, pain, or anxiety of visiting the dentist means a mouth you can be proud of. It also means smiling again—with confidence!

7. **Overwhelmed by thoughts of repeated visits to the dentist?** Maybe you "toughed it out" and got through going to the dentist once—but again? Twice per year? If that thought makes you anxious or even overwhelmed, sedation dentistry can ease your mind and make going to the dentist more of a regular thing.

Hopefully, this chapter has been a huge relief to patients like yourself—patients who feel anxious enough about visiting the dentist to either delay it until it's absolutely necessary or avoid it altogether.

Maybe it's not you who's afraid; maybe it's a son or daughter, your husband or wife, a parent, brother, sister, friend, or neighbor. Regardless of who heeds this advice, heed it well: you don't have to be afraid of going to the dentist any longer. Sedation dentistry is a safe and effective alternative that lets you relax—and even sleep—through your dental visits.

Regardless of who takes advantage of it, sedation dentistry could just be the solution you (or someone you love) have been hoping and praying for. Even if it isn't, don't wait any longer to get the dental care you need. Join the millions of people just like you and experience sedation dentistry's relaxed, easy state where dentistry can be accomplished in just a few visits, in the most comfortable way possible.

Chapter 4:

Cosmetic Dentistry

If you think about it, it all makes perfect sense: poor oral health *is* linked to poor physical health. How so? Well, consider the big picture: your mouth is the gateway into the rest of the body and its various internal systems.

If the mouth has a chronic infection or disease, then your entire body may be indirectly or directly exposed to those bacteria since **everything comes through your mouth**. Not to mention the fact that your ability to eat is compromised, as well as your nutrition.

Furthermore, the valuable physical resources needed for your general health to function—such as energy, metabolism, and white blood cells—will be diverted to handle the chronic infection, weakening the overall natural protection your other systems typically enjoy.

As we have already seen, research documents connections between gum disease and poor heart health, resulting in increased risk of stroke, as well as diabetes, problem pregnancies, respiratory diseases, and certain types of cancers. What's more, some studies indicate that those who lose all their natural teeth may have a much shorter life span.

So what's the answer? If you want to increase your chances of a living happy, healthy life, treat your body with respect and put your money (and effort) where your mouth is. Try starting with the basics: learn the latest tips, techniques, and tools for top-notch oral hygiene when you go in for your next cleaning appointment.

Involve your dental care professional in learning what you can do, in and out of his or her office, to have a cleaner, safer, healthier mouth. Trust me, most dentists would love to hand out more advice, so ask and you shall receive!

Next, branch out: incorporate a healthy diet, proper supplementation (I recommend a professional quality multivitamin supplement, fish oil, CoQ10, pro-biotics and "Juice Plus") exercise, fresh air, and plenty of regular rest. Eliminate unhealthy habits, like smoking and drinking, that are counterproductive to a healthy lifestyle. And remember, taking care of your teeth means better well-being, and it means your body will be better able to take care of itself.

We've covered how easy it is to attend to your routine dental needs, either through regular checkups or sedation dentistry, which can alleviate fear in those patients who experience anxiety about regular checkups. But in this section I want to address those of you for whom a healthy mouth—alone—may not mean true happiness when it comes to your appearance.

A Few Words about Cosmetic Dentistry

Cosmetic dentistry can be technically defined as "the alteration of oral or facial features to correct or enhance a person's smile or oral balance." But in my experience most people who seek cosmetic dentistry are concerned with more than just their appearance; they are seeking an emotional boost, or in some cases are trying to repair emotional damage done by years, or perhaps even a lifetime, of dental imbalance.

Crooked, discolored, missing, or perhaps age-worn teeth can lead people to feel insecure about their smiles; it can even lead to fewer—or no—smiles from traumatized patients. For some, cosmetic dentistry is no more serious than a trip to the beauty salon or tanning bed while for others it can mean a newfound sense of confidence, happiness, and satisfaction they've long missed.

Doing a Self-Smile Analysis

Your smile is one of the first things that other people notice about you. What will they see when you smile? More importantly, what do *you* think they will see? Many patients who come to me seeking cosmetic dentistry are at odds between what they feel about their teeth/smile and what other people see.

There are many ways to analyze your smile. At Imagecare we like to use two different techniques—the emotional evaluation (what you *feel* about how your smile looks) and the objective evaluation (how it really looks). On the following pages is a simple list of questions you can ask yourself to determine the current state of your smile.

Your Pre-Cosmetic Dentistry Objective Evaluation

For the objective analysis, i.e., determining how your smile really looks, the best thing is for you to stand in front of a mirror mounted on a wall. Now, smile at yourself using your "normal" smile. This is the smile you'd give to a friend you meet on the street or a coworker passing in the hall. Next, look at the mirror and think of a hilarious moment in your life and give a great, big, laughing smile.

If you are not happy with your teeth, then this "big" smile is probably a much larger smile than you feel comfortable using much of the time. When your smile is improved, however, your big smile appears much more spontaneously because you look (and feel) great!

So let's figure out what's holding your big smile back from being used more often. In other words, what it is that bothers you about your teeth?

1. Are all of your teeth brilliant white or are they somewhat yellow, dark, or stained?
2. Are there spaces between any of your teeth?
3. Are you missing any of your teeth?
4. Do you have teeth that are crooked, uneven, or otherwise out of line?
5. Do any of your teeth appear short and fat or too small or too large?
6. Are the edges of any of your teeth even with the rest of your teeth, or are they too long or too short?

7. Do your teeth (as a group) slant one way or another?
8. Is the midline of your two front teeth centered with your face and nose?
9. Are the edges of your canine teeth too long, sharp, or out of line?
10. Do you grind your teeth or are any of the biting edges on your teeth chipped or worn down?
11. Do you have a "gummy" smile—i.e. showing too much gum tissue?
12. Are your gums even and in line and symmetrical or irregularly shaped—i.e., higher on some teeth and lower on others?
13. Have your gums receded or do they appear red or puffy?
14. Do you have any gray, black, or silver (mercury) dental fillings in your teeth?
15. Do you have any old crowns that have dark edges at the top or that don't really look natural?

Now that you have taken an objective look at your smile, let's focus on how it makes you feel with what I call an "emotional evaluation."

Your Pre-Cosmetic Dentistry Emotional Evaluation

The emotional smile evaluation is based on each individual's subjective perceptions of his or her smile. In other words, when you smile in the mirror, or simply smile in front of friends or family, how do you "feel" about your smile? Happy? Sad? Proud? Ashamed? Confident? Insecure?

The questions below are designed to help reveal our true inner feelings about how our smile affects our self-image, how it impacts interactions with others, and how it influences the quality of our relationships:

1. Do you love the appearance of your teeth and smile?
2. Do you ever turn your face when smiling or hold your hand up in front of your mouth when talking to others?

3. Have you ever found yourself looking at models or other people with beautiful smiles and wishing you had a similar smile?

4. Have you figured out a way to use your lips to cover any aspect of your smile?

5. Are you embarrassed to visit a cosmetic dentist due to the condition of your teeth or the length of time since your last visit to a dentist?

6. How does your smile make you feel? Confident?

7. Do you shy away from showing a full smile in front of other people, especially strangers?

8. When taking pictures, do you tend to smile with your lips closed instead of flashing a happy smile?

9. Have you ever held back a laugh because you felt uncomfortable about your smile?

10. How would a beautiful new smile make you feel?

11. What would you like to change about your smile?

These questions were designed to help you come to a fair assessment of your smile. If you have any concerns about your smile after this evaluation, speak to a qualified cosmetic dentist to determine if cosmetic dentistry can help you create a smile you truly "feel" great about.

Not sure where or how to find a qualified cosmetic dentist? Don't worry; that's what the rest of this chapter is all about!

Cosmetic Options for Your Smile Makeover

When people hear the words "cosmetic dentistry," they often think of painful, expensive, and prolonged dental treatment; this isn't always the case. Many ancillary items fall under the purview of cosmetic dentistry, to include the following:

- Porcelain veneers
- Invisalign® (Straight teeth without braces)
- Beautiful all-porcelain crowns
- Tooth colored fillings
- Cosmetic bonding

- Tooth recontouring
- Gingival recontouring
- Whitening
- Smile lifts
- Dental implants
- Fuller lips
- Age-defying, younger smiles
- Bioesthetic full mouth rejuvenation
- Comfortable, lifelike dentures and partial denture

Which one—or ones—will be right for you?

This chapter will help you explore a variety of these options, but more importantly, it will help you understand your own needs for seeking cosmetic dentistry, and how knowing yourself better will help you to select the best cosmetic dentist for you.

Eight Essentials for a World-class Cosmetic Dental Makeover: *A Proven System for Successful Smile Makeovers!*

What makes for a classic cosmetic dental makeover? Through years of experience as a cosmetic dentist, advanced training, and completion of over fifty thousand cosmetic restorations, over time I have developed this proven system that produces incredible results time after time:

Essential # 1: *Digital Photos for Imagecare Cosmetic Imaging*

Wouldn't it be great to see what your smile might look like after a procedure is done *before* you get started? Now you can with something called "cosmetic imaging."

Cosmetic dental imaging is crucial so that patients can preview the possibilities before making an investment! During this step of the process your cosmetic dentist will take nine to fifteen pictures of your teeth for smile analysis.

Essential # 2: *Imagecare Smile Analysis*

A "smile analysis" includes data collected about your teeth and how they match up or deviate from what is considered "ideal." In a smile analysis, your cosmetic dentist looks for ways to improve your smile.

Since each one is unique, your dental provider will look at all the factors that compose a smile, such as:

- The shape of your smile
- The size of your teeth
- The smile line
- The position of your teeth, lips, and gums when you smile

After the analysis, you can discuss with your cosmetic dentist what you want to accomplish and any concerns you may have. Once your dentist has this information, he or she can then provide a custom smile design.

Essential # 3: *Imagecare Lip and Gum Analysis*

During the third of these eight steps, your cosmetic dentist will do an evaluation of your gum symmetry and height. Plus, he or she will do a careful evaluation of how your lip line relates to your teeth and how your teeth support your lips. This lip and gum analysis is important because cosmetic dentistry is not just about new teeth, but how those teeth align with, or "fit in with," your lips and gums.

Essential # 4: *Imagecare Bite Analysis (Occlusion)*

Did you know that your teeth don't work individually in your mouth, but instead work together? We call this your "bite," or occlusion. Therefore, a bite analysis is basically an evaluation of the way your teeth function **as a group**.

In fact, a bite analysis is one of the most important aspects of cosmetic dentistry. **Beautiful teeth will not last unless they function right.** And if the forces that caused damage to your teeth in the first place are not addressed, then no matter how good it or your dentist is, your cosmetic dentistry *will* fail.

Essential # 5: *Imagecare New Smile Design*

> *"Perfection is Dr. Thompson's goal, and he achieves it.
> I admire, respect, and appreciate that…A visit
> to Imagecare is always a pleasant experience."*
> **—J.B.**

What's unique about modern dentistry is the amount of visual aids we can use to help patients not only understand the procedures we'll be performing but also how their smile will look when it is done.

Digital photos and your smile analysis are just the beginning; using digital imaging software, your cosmetic dentist will personally generate a custom image, unique to your smile. He or she will review the smile design results with you and discuss how to make it happen.

Essential # 6: *Customized Imagecare Digital Presentation*

> *"Thank you, Dr. Thompson, for giving me a bright new smile.
> I love my porcelain veneers; they look and feel so natural. My new
> look is younger, refreshed, and professional. I can't help but
> smile all the time. Thanks so much!"*
> **—M.W.**

Your dental care professional will prepare for you a custom created PowerPoint presentation showing you what is possible through application of Imagecare New Smile Design principles to your smile.

This is a critical step that allows you and your dentist to be on the exact same page for your new smile. There is real value in you being able to "preview" your new smile and give feedback before you invest any time and money.

It is important for you to know in advance what is possible for your smile. That is why, nowadays, some dental offices have a "smile studio" with state-of-the-art digital photography equipment where your dentist can generate a custom digital image of your smile live, before your very eyes. This is a way of making patients feel comfortable with the "before" and "after" images of what they might look like after their cosmetic procedure.

Essential # 7: *Diagnostic Wax-up Designed by Imagecare*

Seeing your smile "live" and in living color is important for both you and your dental care professional. It's extremely important to have a working model of your desired smile design. This allows your dentist to create prototype (temporary) cosmetic restorations that you will wear while the permanent restorations are being fabricated by a skilled laboratory technician. The goal is to have prototypes so well done that they will mimic the final product.

Consider it a dress rehearsal—for your mouth! This valuable step, our seventh essential for a healthy smile, gives your dentist valuable information and allows for your feedback and correction of problems prior to receiving permanent restorations

Essential # 8: *World-class Laboratory Work*

Depending on the size of the dental practice, the various products and appliances used in your cosmetic procedure are typically created in-house or sent to an outside lab.

When sent to an outside lab, the laboratory technician must be a highly trained and skilled craftsman. It takes a ceramic artist to defy nature and provide long-lasting natural beauty. It is common today for some dental labs to outsource your restorations to other countries, so *beware*!

Always feel free to ask your dentist for more information about his or her laboratory technicians to make sure you're getting the best quality possible. Remember, it's *your* mouth!

How to Be Sure Your Cosmetic Dentist Is the "Real Deal"

Any dentist who has graduated from a dental school can call him or herself a "cosmetic" dentist, but is he or she really qualified to do cosmetic dentistry? In other words, dentists don't have to have any special training in cosmetic dentistry in order to legally call themselves "cosmetic dentists."

But! There *are* dentists out there who have been trained specifically in cosmetic procedures. These dentists are *true* cosmetic dentists who possess a winning combination of a foundation in general dentistry and the artistic training to give you the cosmetic smile makeover you're looking for.

One of the major differences between a "general" dentist and a cosmetic dentist is this: a cosmetic dentist has a strong esthetic eye, and is dedicated to continuing education in the field of cosmetic dentistry. He or she also specializes in several types of cosmetic dentistry and is proficient in his or her "niche" markets.

So, how else can *you* tell the difference between the two so you can make sure you don't end up with a less qualified cosmetic dentist?

Here's how: in addition to asking for before-and-after photos and checking references (as we mentioned above), check to see if your cosmetic dentist is a member of the American Academy of Cosmetic Dentistry (AACD).

The AACD is an organization of cosmetic dentists who are committed to the highest levels of education and advancement in the area of cosmetic dentistry. In fact, the AACD is made up of an elite, highly trained group of cosmetic dentists from around the world!

If you can find a cosmetic dentist who is a member of the AACD, chances are they specialize in cosmetic dentistry, which means it most likely makes up the bulk of the treatments they provide...

And full-time cosmetic dentists will have performed many procedures that will have allowed them to hone their skills and perfect their techniques—leaving you with ideal results!

Here's another secret: make sure you find a cosmetic dentist who is a fellow and a master in the Academy of General Dentistry! This advanced certification proves that your dentist has spent hundreds of additional hours of continuing education to deliver the best cosmetic dentistry.

One other important tip: this will be hard to find, but if you can locate a cosmetic dentist who has graduated from Levels 1, 2, 3, *and* 4 of the OBI Foundation for Bioesthetic Dentistry, then you will know **without a doubt** that you have found a dentist who has had some of the most intense and thorough training in the world! This is more than just a regular dentist; this person is an authority on esthetics and occlusion (bite).

The reason this is so important is that, in my opinion, a large percentage of cosmetic dentistry performed on worn or chipped teeth is actually only a cover-up for undiagnosed occlusal (bite) disharmony. You have got to find a dentist that knows how to definitively solve these problems at the root source, and not just cover them up—or patch them—using the latest techniques.

Last but not least, it could be essential to you that your cosmetic dentist has an advanced understanding of orthodontics because some cosmetic cases require tooth movement with or without braces to give you that WOW smile! Be sure to inquire about your dentist's experience in/with orthodontics before making any definitive choice.

Does Age Matter? Surprisingly, Not When It Comes to Cosmetic Dentistry

I feel that any adult regardless of age is a candidate for cosmetic dentistry. In fact, age should never be a factor in choosing cosmetic dentistry. It is never too late for a younger looking smile. A recently released nationwide survey concluded that an attractive smile has a positive impact on relationships, both professional and personal.

For these reasons and many others, people are seeking brighter, younger smiles in record numbers. Improving your smile with cosmetic dentistry is a wonderful solution for those who want to make a great first impression.

It has been shown that an improved smile can boost a person's self-confidence. And if you're confident about your smile, chances are you'll smile more. And a smiling face is more friendly and positive. Charles Gordy once said, "A smile is an inexpensive way to change your looks."

The treatment needed to rejuvenate a smile varies. For some people it may be as simple as teeth whitening or updating to esthetic fillings, crowns, or veneers. But for those with severely worn or stained teeth, it could require a complete mouth rejuvenation. The great news is that many smiles can be dramatically improved in just a few appointments!

In an age where everyone values the gift of an attractive smile, people of all ages can have the smile they always dreamed of. Cosmetic dentistry can change your smile, and it just might change your life!

Porcelain Veneers: *The Workhorse of Cosmetic Dentistry*

Many people dream of having a brighter, cleaner, more attractive smile, but in reality they have chipped, stained, discolored, unevenly spaced, or even slightly crooked front teeth. In many cases, porcelain veneers are the *perfect* solution to address these issues safely and affordably.

Veneers are one of the most versatile restoration options available on the market today, providing a completely new-looking smile or restoring an aged, possibly even worn smile to its original beauty. For a qualified dental professional, applying porcelain veneers is a simple process involving bonding thin, contact lens–like coverings to the teeth.

The versatility of veneers designed by your cosmetic dentist allows him or her to create more attractive tooth size color or shape. And in many cases, veneers can provide a long-lasting, stain-resistant alternative to crowns.

If you *are* interested in porcelain veneers or any cosmetic procedure, you can always schedule a complimentary consultation with your dentist. What happens then? Your cosmetic dentist will first carefully evaluate your specific situation, and listen while you explain the exact changes you have in mind.

He or she will then show you some pictures of similar smiles that have undergone this type of transformation. Then comes the exciting part—this is where skill and experience comes in: your dentist will take digital photographs of your existing teeth and smile.

Your cosmetic dentist will then apply cosmetic smile design principles while he or she artistically recreates your smile with digital imaging. A special Power Point presentation may even be offered by some dental offices, allowing you to see just what is possible—in living color!

People are always curious about what their dentist can do to enhance their smile. A qualified dental care provider can always visualize a patient's new smile because he or she will have done so many of these makeovers. And, of course, describing those changes verbally, seeing other patients' smiles in a photo album or even seeing a wax-up model of your teeth helps, but it isn't adequate.

Imaging is a powerful tool that allows your dentist to communicate with you, visually, what a new smile can do for you. It's not only professionally helpful to aid in the "smile design" process, but also personally helpful to aid in the patient's understanding of the process itself. Plus it's just fun for the patients to see the changes on themselves!

Once you're ready to begin treatment, your dentist will take an impression of your mouth for a "diagnostic wax up," giving you a three-dimensional representation of the results. The wax-up will guide your dental care provider in preparation of the teeth and will serve as a template for your temporary (prototype) veneers.

Often, porcelain veneers can provide a completely improved and dazzling smile in just a few appointments. The actual treatment usually involves only two visits. The number of preoperative visits depends on the complexity of your situation and the changes you desire.

There usually is a follow-up visit or two for final adjustments (engineering checks) and polishing. Specific and detailed instructions will be given for care of your new smile to insure it lasts years and years.

Parting Words for the Worried: *How to Recession Proof Your (Cosmetic) SMILE*

In uncertain economic times, it is important not only to maintain your smile but to ensure it does not become a liability. We all agree that having to buy a root canal and crown is about as exciting as having to buy new tires for your car or an unexpected expensive household repair.

So with uncertain times ahead, wouldn't it make sense to recession proof your smile? It's actually very easy; here's how:

- **Prevention, prevention, prevention.** Stay current with your biannual cleaning, X-rays, and exams. Prevention and early detection is the best way to minimize dental expenses.

- **Maximize use of insurance benefits and medical savings accounts.** Remember that unused benefits do not roll over. So don't leave any benefits on the table!

- **Block out decay.** Let your hygienist know that you want a fluoride treatment. Fluoride reinforces your enamel against tooth decay and helps prevent costly cavities!

- **Get necessary treatment completed.** Dental problems left untreated will only get worse and more expensive to correct. Furthermore, they will often result in painful emergency situations usually at the worst of times. (Murphy's Law!)

- **Identify all potential problems to avoid surprises.** Make sure that your dentist identifies all potential problems such as old mercury fillings, old crowns, and wisdom teeth. There are often hidden problems lurking under these old restorations prone to cause expensive dental work.

- **Make sure you get a warranty!** If you do need dental work, such as a crown, make sure your new crown comes with a warranty. Experienced and reputable dentists will usually guarantee their work.

- **Finally, protect your assets.** Wear a custom-made night guard. A properly made night guard will protect your teeth from nighttime clenching and grinding forces that can damage or destroy dental restorations, bone support, and gum health.

Cosmetic dentistry shouldn't be avoided merely because of price concerns. Hopefully some of these tips will help you afford cosmetic dentistry sooner to help avoid dental problems later!

Chapter 5

Dental Implants

Once upon a time, back in the (very) early days of dentistry, lost teeth truly were "lost," and even those who weren't happy with the placement, gaps, or size of their teeth were essentially stuck with what they had. Fortunately, this is no longer the case. Thanks to modern technology and the rise of dental implants, you don't have to be satisfied with an unsatisfactory smile any longer.

When permanent teeth are lost, regardless of the reason or number of teeth, dental implants can offer a "new lease on life." They are often superior to other choices because they are solid, secure, and esthetic (i.e., they look good). If you're worried about safety or permanence, don't. After nearly thirty-five years of use, dental implants have a 90–95 percent proven success rate in appropriately chosen cases.

Dental Implants: *Permanent, Secure, Tooth Replacements*

What, exactly, is a dental implant?

An implant is a special surgical grade titanium post, manufactured to highly precise specifications, under strict sterile conditions, that is inserted surgically into the jawbone below the gum surface. Sounds serious, right? And painful? Relax; with proper use of the newest anesthetics and medications, you need not be concerned about pain.

As the bone bonds to the post, it forms a secure foundation onto which your new teeth are then attached and shaped to match your mouth. The number of teeth being replaced will determine the best kind of restoration for you.

Implants can help replace a single tooth or a full set of teeth. If you have been suffering with partial or full dentures, are missing teeth, or feel you need teeth extracted, do not hesitate to call a properly trained implant dentist to be evaluated for implants, which can literally give you—and your mouth—a new lease on life.

The Advantages of a Dental Implant

Dental implants have a variety of benefits.

- **They are permanent.** A dental implant is not a denture that can be taken in and out of your mouth; it is permanent and secure. Implants often anchor permanent or removable dentures.

- **They are convenient.** You won't have to take your dental implant out before a meal.

- **There is no messy cleanup.** You won't have to buy and use expensive, messy powders, gels, or tablets to clean your implants with. You can brush, floss, and care for them as you would your natural teeth.

- **They are compatible with your existing, natural teeth.** Modern dental implants can be made to look like the rest of your teeth.

- **They won't look like "false" teeth.** In fact, great care is taken to match the color and the shade of your dental implant so that there isn't the slightest hint of it being a false tooth.

- **The implants are placed into the jawbone.** They "integrate" securely and help prevent bone loss in areas where there are missing teeth.

- **A dental implant is stand-alone and does not need to depend on the adjoining teeth for support like a dental bridge.** This is of primary importance. When the surrounding teeth are healthy, they don't have to be ground down like they would for a bridge.

- **They are extremely comfortable.**

- **They provide a source of confidence.** With secure dental implants you can step out in style and confidence, completely satisfied that this was a good decision.

Implant Placement

After determining that implants are for you, and having a thorough examination by your dentist, the next step is actually placing the implant in the jaw. While it may sound serious, this routine procedure is normally carried out under local anesthesia in the dental office.

When the procedure is completed, the implant is left to integrate naturally to the bone. As you might imagine, it takes approximately eight to twelve weeks for the healthy bone to form a strong bond and fuse with the implant.

In order to qualify for a dental implant, you need to be healthy and not be suffering from any significant physical ailments. The dentist will need to check the amount of healthy bone available, the condition of your gums, and make sure that you do not suffer from periodontal disease. If not, then there is no need to delay the restoration of missing teeth. Dental implants are safe, secure, and best of all give you the confidence to smile again!

Taking Care of Your Dental Implant

Now that you've gotten dental implants, the best thing you can do to preserve and enjoy them is to start taking care of them right away. Just like your "regular" teeth, a dental implant needs to be part of your daily normal oral hygiene. Ensure that you brush and floss twice a day so that there is no chance of infection or for bacteria to accumulate.

Your implant dentist will develop the best care plan for you. Follow it thoroughly. Do not miss the appointments that have been scheduled. This way your dentist will be in a position to make sure that both your teeth and gums remain strong and in good shape.

If you are considering dental implants, clearly there is a world of opportunity out there affording you the latest in dental care and implant technology. Regardless of whether or not you choose a dental implant, don't let cost, coverage, or concern stop you from obtaining the mouth—and the smile—you were born to get.

As we have seen throughout this chapter, there is always a personal alternative that's right for you; you just have to seek out patient centered dental care and make sure you know what you're getting into first.

This chapter was meant to empower you—with facts, information, and logic—to face your smile issues head on and without fear. Now that you know how simple, safe, and dependable dental implants can be, don't hesitate to contact your local dentist about choosing the option that's right for you!

Chapter 6:

All About Invisalign

When it comes to "getting your smile on," most of us picture a set of straight, white, evenly spaced teeth. However, that smile eludes most of us. In fact, many of my patients grew up with crooked or widely spaced teeth that never got "fixed" during childhood or even young adulthood.

Those patients, combined with patients who did have braces as youths and now have had relapses, make up a large part of the esthetic concerns that many of my patients have. There is simply no reason to avoid solving these issues now that you're an adult.

Why? Invisalign clear braces provide patients with a revolutionary way to straighten teeth without the limitations of traditional braces. Now, you can choose to improve the look and function of your teeth with flexible, removable Invisalign braces.

Even adults who wore braces as children can often find themselves in need of Invisalign later in life. Maybe their teeth have "relapsed," leaving one or two crooked, or perhaps they have become too crowded over time and things are getting worse. These affordable clear braces for teens *and* adults can be the solution you're looking for.

Invisalign Removes the Embarrassment of Braces

The world of orthodontia has definitely taken a turn for the better in recent years. Never again will you need to be embarrassed to show off your smile while wearing braces! Invisalign has become the darling of the dental world, and celebrities are at the top of the list of those clamoring to wear them.

Since public image and the ability to look good in a close-up are vital to the survival of the careers of public figures, anything that will improve their looks while not drawing negative attention is always sought. In other words, celebrities definitely do not want to be caught dead in metal braces!

Invisalign is so chic that even celebrities like actress Kathryn Heigl and supermodel Giselle Bundchen think they are "cool" and have been photographed while secretly wearing Invisalign, while no one was the wiser. It's been widely rumored that Tom Cruise and even Oprah have worn Invisalign (rumored, since no one could tell they had them on!). With Invisalign, their smile is always ready for a close-up, even while wearing braces!

But the good news is you don't have to be famous to take advantage of the many benefits of Invisalign.

Invisalign—Not Just for the Rich and Famous

Although celebrities are the most photographed, and probably the most vain, "fans" of Invisalign, everyone wants to be attractive and have the self-confidence that comes with a beautiful smile. The corporate executive wants to be confident that he or she looks their best when confronting a room full of board members. The soccer mom wants to look good so her family will be proud to show her off to friends.

Teenagers, who already have enough angst and insecurity in their lives, don't want the humiliation of ridicule from wearing metal braces. And, of course, singles don't want to tackle the grueling world of dating while they have metal appliances in their mouth—it takes a lot of the romance away.

Since Invisalign's invention in 1997, hundreds of thousands of "everyday" people can attest to the wonders of this remarkable advance in technology. Why are so many people turning to Invisalign? I think once you see how it works, you'll see why these clear braces are so popular:

How Invisalign Works

Invisalign uses a series of clear removable "aligners" (pictured below) to straighten your teeth without metal wires or brackets. The aligners work together so that, in a prescribed series, they slowly but noticeably change the alignment of your teeth (hence their name). So you don't just get one aligner but a series of aligners—ranging from fifteen to twenty-five total—that your dentist will instruct you how to use, and when, for maximum effectiveness.

Although the Invisalign aligners aren't for everyone, over 80 percent of people *can* wear them. Only your dentist can determine that for certain, and the first step is an evaluation of your needs and personal circumstances.

How does it work? After a 3-D computerized analysis is completed, treatment goals are established for your individual situation. Your unique situation will determine the type of treatment course to take.

The "express" treatment course is structured for those with lesser problems and a shortened program. You may only need ten aligners or less, with less overall time to make the corrections.

The "regular" treatment involves wearing your clear, plastic aligners for approximately twenty-three hours a day from two to twenty-four months. Approximately every two weeks, after your teeth have fit perfectly into the aligners, you will replace those aligners with new ones—and the process will continue. Every six weeks you will meet with your dentist to have your progress checked.

During the intervals you will have the flexibility of removing the aligners to eat, drink coffee or alcohol, brush, floss—and for a romantic interlude if you want. Keep in mind that the longer you wear your aligners the more effective they will be.

Invisalign: *It's All About the 5 C's*

There are numerous advantages to wearing the clear Invisalign aligners. The five main ones are what I call "the 5 C's," which include:

- **Confidence**: Invisalign helps improve your physical appearance, which in turn promotes healthy self-esteem.
- **Comfort**: Invisalign is painless, making it very comfortable.
- **Concealment**: Invisibility is one of the reasons my patients love Invisalign.

- **Culture**: Invisalign fits with your modern lifestyle.
- **Cost**: Affordability makes Invisalign extremely popular.

Now that you know what the 5 C's are, let's learn a little more about each one.

Confidence

People who have crooked teeth, gaps between their teeth, or other noticeable and unsightly tooth problems are usually self-conscious. They may cover up their mouths with their hands, bite their lips, or even avoid smiling altogether. Some people who are insecure about their smiles are mistaken for being rude or shy, and often are avoided by others. This is one case where a physical problem can quickly turn emotional.

A mouth with straight teeth allows them to open up and exude the confidence and positive self-image they have been without, oftentimes for years on end. A person with a bright and open smile makes a good impression, and opens doors to some remarkable opportunities that may not have been available before.

Comfort

The Invisalign aligners are nearly painless. Although there may be a slight sense of discomfort at the beginning of the process (which is natural as patients—and their teeth—get accustomed to the aligners), they are nowhere near as painful as old-fashioned metal braces. What's more, you will no longer experience the ulcerated gums, wires poking into your skin, or rubber bands snapping in your mouth once associated with wire braces.

There also is the advantage of fewer appointments needed with the Invisalign. What would have taken two years with traditional braces can often be accomplished in far less time with the clear aligners, and with fewer visits to the dentist to disrupt your schedule.

Concealment

Since Invisalign is comprised of two clear aligners—one on your top row of teeth and one on the bottom, they are virtually camouflaged in your mouth. You can wear them at work or play, and unless you point them out to someone they will usually not be detected.

You can also avoid the mental anguish and embarrassment associated with wearing metal braces—and the cruel remarks passing as jokes when someone draws attention to you with terms like "metal mouth," "tin grin," or "brace face."

Some people do not want others to know they are wearing braces, for whatever reason. With Invisalign your privacy is concealed. You only have to expose your secret if you want to—or perhaps when the results are "clear"!

Culture

There is no disruption of your lifestyle while undergoing treatment. You do not have to remove your Invisalign aligners to work out at the gym or even speak in public. You do not have to avoid certain food or drink, you can speak without slurring, and you can take the aligners out if you absolutely need to for special occasions.

You also take the plastic aligners out when you eat, drink, and brush your teeth. There is no worry that food will get caught in these braces, and you can eat apples, caramel, and other sticky foods without anything getting caught in wires–even kiss another person without sticking them with your braces.

Cost

In the long run, your particular plan of treatment will determine the actual cost. With Invisalign you can almost guarantee that you will be saved years of time and pain, and possibly thousands of dollars. Your dentist and his staff will work with you to fit your plan into your budget.

For those patients in need of assistance, financing through Care Credit, a third-party health care financing company that offers monthly payments, with no annual fees, prepayment penalties, or upfront costs, is available. It's also possible that your insurance company will cover a portion of your orthodontic treatment.

Teen Treatment: *Will My Kids Go for Invisalign?*

Since teens are especially vulnerable to ridicule and peer pressure, Invisalign offers so many positive alternatives to traditional braces that the possibility of their use can't be ignored.

The fact that celebrities think they are "cool" is definitely a plus, but nothing is more important than making vital corrections to dental health early, while the cost is less and vital adjustments are made before any damage from incoming wisdom teeth or jaw problems go untreated.

As an added bonus for parents, six free aligners are included in your teen's course of treatment, and a special blue button is inserted in a teen's aligners that will allow the dentist to keep track of whether the teen is complying with the treatment or not. This will help keep the treatment on track and ensure the parents' investment.

Ten Simple Dental Care Tips While Using Invisalign

"What's it like to wear Invisalign?"

"Will I have to take care of my teeth differently?"

"Will they hurt?"

"Will I get bad breath?"

These are just a few of the very logical, very common questions I get each week from people interested in using Invisalign clear braces. So to answer them in print, I've listed below ten simple dental care tips while using Invisalign:

1. **Always brush your teeth twice a day.** Brush your teeth twice a day to avoid majority of the dental problems. Brushing incorrectly may reduce its effectiveness. It's important to know *how to correctly brush your teeth*.

2. **Use dental floss twice a day.** Flossing cleans the areas that are harder for a toothbrush to reach. It removes the food debris and plaque accumulated between the teeth. Flossing twice daily is preferable.

3. **Use mouthwash to kill bacterial plaque.** Mouthwashes such as Listerine or Chlorohexidine possess effective anti-

septic properties. They kill the bacterial plaque known to cause bad breath, tooth decay, and gingivitis. Use a mouthwash *after* brushing as per its directions.

4. **Eat right.** Maintain a balanced diet but reduce the consumption of foods containing sugars or starch. Sugary foods (candies, gums) and starchy foods (potato chips, snacks) play an important role in causing tooth decay.

5. **Avoid in-between eating habits.** Snacking between meals makes teeth prone to tooth decay. The bacterial action is greatest at acidic pH. The pH is most acidic immediately after meals, and then gradually reduces and comes to a normal level. Eating in between meals does not allow the acidic level to come down, increasing bacterial action leading to cavities.

6. **Avoid cola and energy drinks.** Cola drinks contain acids such as phosphoric acid and citric acid, which have damaging effect on teeth. Energy drinks contain organic acids in addition to the above, which directly damage the tooth calcium. **Energy drinks and commercial lemonade are eleven times more harmful to teeth than cola drinks.** If you must drink, don't sip on them for a long time and do rinse your mouth after drinking.

7. **Quit smoking.** Smoking not only stains your teeth but also damages your gums by reducing the blood supply. It also causes smoker's breath.

8. **Avoid chewing gum.** Chewing gum will damage or cause the aligners to become dislodged.

9. **Continue with regular visits to your dentist.** It is essential to visit your dentist once every three to six months to diagnose any oral concerns early. Most oral health problems do not produce any symptoms till they have progressed to a later stage.

10. **Remove or avoid oral piercings:** Oral piercings such as tongue or lip are a no-no for good oral health. Tongue piercings can lead to allergic reactions, infections, nervous damage to tongue, and gum disease.

How to Choose an Invisalign Dentist Who's Right for You!

At some time or another you will be faced with looking for a new dentist. Like most people, you want to find a dentist you can trust, who will care for you and your family, and who has your best interests in mind.

Since this is an important decision in your life, I have decided to give you "**The Inside Scoop on How to Choose a Dentist That's Right for You!**" to help guide you to the right dentist. I have seen so many people in pain and suffer mentally and financially throughout my years in practice simply because of poor dental work. Most people don't know how to go about selecting a dentist, or even realize the problems that can occur if you don't choose wisely. Together, we are not going to let that happen to you.

- **Tip #1:** Ask for recommendations. Go to review Web sites such as www.doctoroogle.com to read reviews concerning the dentist in consideration.

- **Tip #2:** Check the dentist's license and credentials. It may sound simplistic but check with the dental board in your state for license status and if any disciplinary action has been taken against that dentist. Credentials are huge in dentistry! Make sure your dentist is a fellow or a master in the Academy of General Dentistry (FAGD) (www.agd.org). This credential alone is worth its weight in gold, as you know that a "fellowed" dentist is committed to lifelong learning and staying current with the latest treatment techniques to keep you comfortable and safe. Make sure your Invisalign dentist has completed Invisalign Clear Essentials 1 and 2 training courses and has stayed current on evolving Invisalign treatment protocol.

- **TIP #3:** Ask for verification of diagnosis. It is critical that you find a dentist who has digital X-rays so you can see on the computer screen. Most dentists with integrity will show you your X-rays but sometimes, even better, a great dentist will show you an intraoral camera picture of your teeth so you will know exactly what the doctor sees in your mouth. Seeing this opens great communication about your condition, your options, and allows you to be a part of deciding your dental treatment!

- **Tip #4:** Visit the office or take advantage of a free consultation! Look for a courteous staff and a doctor that listens and takes the time to answer your questions.

- **Tip #5:** Ask the right questions. This is a big one since most patients don't know the critical questions to ask. Ask about infection control (especially with the H1N1 spreading)! Does the office follow the recently updated CDC guidelines? Do they participate in a program to monthly monitor the effectiveness of their sterilizers? Ask about staff training. Are the dental assistants and hygienist current with CPR, nitrous oxide monitoring, and X-ray techniques? Ask about insurance. Does the office in consideration help you file your insurance and make every effort to be up-front and answer your questions regarding scheduling and billing? Does the office have a payment plan in place?

- **Tip #6:** Observe the chair-side manner of the doctor/hygienist. Does your doctor/hygienist take time to listen to you, make eye contact, and have a sympathetic, caring manner? What about personality? Going to the dentist is stressful enough; you want someone who is warm, friendly, has a great sense of humor, and puts you at ease! You want an office where you can connect and feel at home.

Now that we have given you the insider information on how to find the right dentist for you and your family, it is time for you to take action. Please don't delay dental care! We want you to be healthy, happy about your smile, and pain free for life!

Conclusion:

Now, Go Get Your Smile On!

Congratulations!

Now you know the answers to the six most commonly asked questions of dentists all over the country. So...how does it feel? Are you more certain than ever that having the smile you've always wanted is just in reach?

I hope so. I wrote this book not just for my own patients but also for patients all over the world. No one needs to suffer through a crooked, awkward, embarrassing, or even painful smile; there is just no excuse.

Now more than ever your local dentist has the tools he or she needs to perform the procedures you want. From regular cleanings and checkups to chronic pain associated with TMJ to cosmetic dentistry, dental implants, and Invisalign—and everything in between—if your regular dentist can't help you, someone locally can.

Take this book to heart; learn its lessons and take charge of your smile. Yes, absolutely, books like this can help, and so can hundreds of Web sites all over the Internet, but until you make that call and find the dentist that is right for you, that perfect smile will always elude you.

Don't let it. This is probably more than you've ever known about dentistry in one sitting! I get that. But it's for a reason: you picked this book up because you had questions. Maybe one, maybe two, maybe all six!

Either way, now you know the answers to your questions and you *can* do something about it. The time is now; don't wait another day to get in touch with your dentist and tell him or her you're ready. For what? Why, ready to *get your smile on*, of course!

By the way don't forget to download your free bonus chapter: Are Dermal Fillers and Botox Right for You? Botox and Dermal Fillers are safe and effective way to get rid of unwanted wrinkles and lines. Or maybe your thinking about fuller lips to further enhance your smile? Go ahead its easy, just type in www. GetYourSmileOnBook.com/bonus-chapter. If you are interested in Imagecare helping you with any of your dental needs, look for the coupon page at the end of this book for some special offers.

About the Author

Dr. Steve Thompson DDS, MAGD
Master of the Academy of General Dentistry

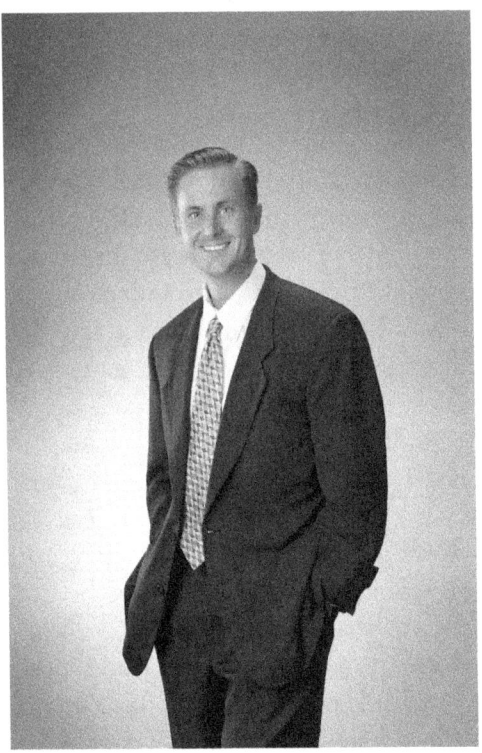

My name is Dr. Steve Thompson, and I have practiced dentistry in Plano, Texas, since 1994. I am often asked, "Why in the world did you want to become a dentist?" Well, here is my story.

Years ago in 1966, I was born in the panhandle of Texas in a small town called Borger (about a two hour drive north of Amarillo) amid big oil refineries, natural gas refineries, and carbon black plants. You may think that all the pollution spewing into the air must have affected my brain cells and altered my DNA, causing me to become a dentist! Who knows, maybe there is some truth to that! Shortly thereafter we moved to Lubbock, Texas.

It is there that I have some of my earliest memories as a child. I remember my dad's big blue Chevy truck, sycamore trees lining the driveway, and the layout and specific trees in our backyard. It's funny, though, that I don't have any memories of the inside of the house, where I'm sure I spent most of my time.

Moving on from Lubbock after a brief stay, we landed in Greenville, Texas. When people ask me where I'm from, I always say Greenville, Texas. It was there that I began to "train" for the dental profession. From when I was old enough to walk and hold a screwdriver, my parents have told me that I loved taking things apart and at least "trying" to put them back together.

As I grew older I loved to draw, build model airplanes, fix lawnmowers, build tree houses and forts, soup up go-karts and became known as a kid who could "fix anything." And I would always fix everything with flare and style. Not only did I fix things, I had to make them look great or I just wasn't happy inside.

The art lessons my parents "made me take" and that I soon learned to enjoy helped me to realize that order, balance, and natural beauty were critical to creating a masterpiece. I believe all this training helped me with my manual dexterity, critical thinking, hand eye coordination, and artistic eye for beautiful smiles, on which I rely on a daily basis.

When I wasn't fixing things you could most certainly find me delivering newspapers or running my lawn-mowing business. I formed my first business at about the age of thirteen with a friend and called it T&H Lawn Mowing service. We even made business cards! I still remember them; they were hand typed on a manual typewriter with red construction paper. It was during these years that I learned about delivering quality service at a fair price, exceptional customer service, and all the basics of how to run a successful small business. I knew from an early age I was destined to be a self-employed small business owner.

After high school in Greenville, I attended East Texas State for a semester studying computer science and began a work-study program at E-Systems, a defense contracting company. Even though I enjoyed programming, I knew that this wasn't what I was called to do, so I decided to join the Army National Guard. I knew this would be a great opportunity to serve my country; the G.I. Bill would help me with college tuition and give me some time to decide what I wanted to do in life.

After returning from boot camp and advanced training, the door was opened for me to attend Texas A&M University. Gig 'em, Aggies!! I really enjoyed A&M, and after my third year I was accepted into Baylor College of Dentistry, from which I graduated with honors in 1994.

Dentistry has been a great fit for me, and I really enjoy being a dentist. I have a real passion for cosmetic and implant dentistry, plus I enjoy helping people with TMJ pain, bad bites, and age-worn smiles. My goal for Imagecare Dental is to educate our patients, and for all our patients to receive expert dental care combined with outstanding customer service. We want to help you achieve optimal oral health!

Oh, I almost forgot, one last thing: *Get Your Smile On!*

www.GetYourSmileOnBook.com/Free-Gift